WIN THE ALK POSITIVE LUNG CANCER FIGHT

STOP TUMOR GROWTH, EXTEND MAXIMUM SURVIVAL USING TARGETED THERAPY, MINIMIZE SIDE EFFECTS, ACHIEVE BREAK THROUGH RESULTS WITH CUTTING EDGE TECHNOLOGY OF PRECISION MEDICINE

DR. PREETAM JAIN

ABOUT THE AUTHOR

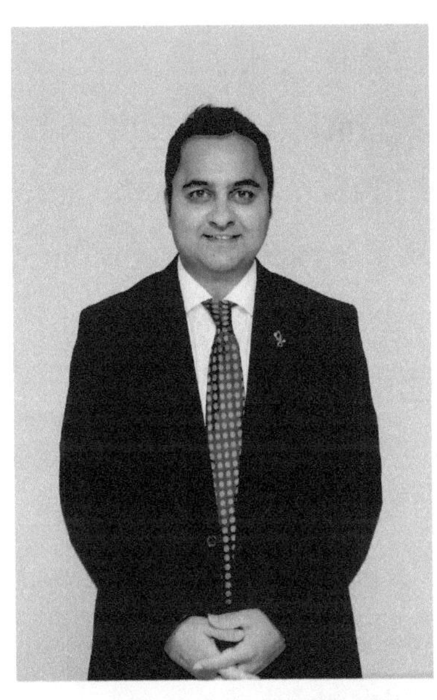

Dr. Preetam Jain, MD, DM, ECMO, is an eminent Medical Oncologist and consultant at leading hospitals in Mumbai, India. With over 15 years of experience, his journey is marked by academic brilliance, unwavering commitment to patient care, and outstanding contributions to oncology, particularly in lung cancer treatment. A gold medalist with distinction, Dr. Jain has earned multiple awards, including the Healthcare Excellence Award, Excellence in Oncology in the Indian Health

Award, Outstanding Young Achievement Award, and Social Impact Award. His book:

"Win The ALK-Positive Lung Cancer Fight"

"Stop Tumor Growth, Extend Maximum Survival using Targeted Therapy, Minimize Side Effects, Achieve Break Through Results with Cutting Edge Technology of Precision Medicine"

His dedication to providing knowledge, hope, and empowerment to lung cancer patients and their families. Driven by a deep sense of compassion and a personal commitment to improving patient outcomes, Dr. Jains approach combines cutting-edge medical science with genuine empathy. His dedication to his craft and his commitment to helping others look and feel their best have earned him a reputation as one of the most trusted and respected Medical Oncologists in the industry. Looking to the future, Dr. Jain remains committed to advancing cancer care, with the goal of improving not only survival rates but the overall Quality of life for his patients. His patient-first philosophy ensures that every individual receives the best possible treatment, along with the emotional and psychological support needed throughout their journey. Besides his professional achievements,

Dr. Jain has a passion for traveling and is known for his exceptional oratory skills. A keen cricket player and an avid socializer, he delights in connecting with friends and colleagues. His active participation in social events and networking opportunities highlights his innate charm and grace, making him a charismatic presence both personally and professionally.

instagram.com/preetamjain_oncologist_mumbai/profilecard/

linkedin.com/in/preetam-kumar-jain-6001b656

CONTENTS

The Introduction

The ALK Villain and the Heroes Fighting Back

In the world of ALK-positive lung cancer, there's a sneaky villain named ALK (Anaplastic Lymphoma Kinase). This troublemaker hides in the cells, causing chaos by making tumors grow. But don't worry—there are powerful superheroes in the form of ALK inhibitors, specialized treatments designed to stop the villain in its tracks. Alongside these heroes are the health detectives—Medical Oncologist and Scientists who use advanced tools and techniques to track down ALK and figure out how to beat it. Together, they're in a constant battle to outsmart the villain and bring hope to patients. Let us dive deep into the understanding of ALK-positive lung cancer.

CHAPTER 1

— ◆ —

UNDERSTANDING ALK POSITIVE LUNG CANCER

Definition, Meaning, and Location

Understanding ALK-Positive Lung Cancer: A Friendly Guide

Hey FOLKS! Let's talk about something called ALK-positive lung cancer. I know it sounds complicated, but don't worry—**we'll break it down together.**

Q) What's This ALK-Positive Lung Cancer All About?

Imagine your lungs are like a busy city. In a healthy city, everything runs smoothly. But sometimes, a troublemaker shows up and causes chaos. In **ALK-positive lung cancer**, that troublemaker is a mixup in a **gene called ALK.**

Q) What's ALK? It Sounds Like a Text Message Abbreviation!

ALK stands for **Anaplastic Lymphoma Kinase.** I know it's a mouthful! **Let's break it down:**

- **Anaplastic**: Think of cells gone rebel, not following the rules.

- **Lymphoma**: This word usually talks about blood cancers, but our ALK troublemaker can cause mischief in lung cells, too.

- **Kinase**: This is like a messenger in your body, passing along signals that tell cells what to do.

So **ALK is basically a protein** that's supposed to help your cells communicate. But when it **goes haywire, it can lead to cancer.**

Q) Where's This ALK Hiding?

Good question! **Imagine ALK is like a book in the library of your body:**

1. The 'story' of ALK (the gene) is written on **chromosome 2** in your DNA.

2. Usually, the ALK protein hangs out on the surface of some cells, like a guard watching for signals.

3. But in ALK-positive lung cancer, it's like two books got mixed up. The ALK 'story' gets jumbled with another gene's story. This creates a troublemaker protein that's always yelling "Grow! Grow!" to your cells.

4. These confused cells usually start causing trouble in your lungs. But if not caught early, they can be like tourists and travel to other parts of your body.

Q) Why Is This Important to Know?

Understanding ALK-positive lung cancer is like having a map of the enemy's base. It helps the oncologist figure out the best way to attack the problem. They can use special medicines that target this mixed-up ALK protein wherever it's hiding in the body.

Remember, knowledge is power. The more we understand about this tricky customer, the better we can fight it. And that's exactly what oncologist and researchers are doing every day!

Q) The ALK-Positive Cancer Story: When Genes Get Mixed Up

Some scientists by the name Soda et al discovered **the EML4-ALK fusion back in 2007.** It's called **"ALK-positive cancer,"** and it's got a pretty interesting story.

Q) When the Gene Tango Gone Wrong

Imagine your DNA as a massive library, with genes as books. Now, in 2007, scientists noticed something odd—two books in this library were getting mixed up. These books were called **EML4 and ALK** (anaplastic lymphoma kinase—quite a mouthful, right?)

Q) What is EML + ALK Fusion: The Trouble-making Duo?

When these two gene 'books' get shuffled together, they create what scientists call a "fusion oncogene." Fancy term alert! But don't worry, it's just a way of saying these mixed-up genes can cause trouble—the kind of trouble that might lead to cancer.

Q) So what's the big deal?

When the **ALK gene gets rearranged** (or mixed up), it's like a **faulty traffic light**. Instead of telling cells when to stop growing, it's stuck on "go, go, go!" This non-stop growth signal is what can lead to cancer.

Q) Has the ALK Rearrangement Cell Party Gone Wild?

If you hear your Oncologist talking about an "ALK re-arrangement," they're basically saying part of your ALK gene has gone rogue. It's like a DJ at a cell party who won't stop the music–the cells keep dancing (or, in this case, multiplying) out of control.

Q) Why does this ALK-positive lung cancer matter?

Understanding this gene mix-up is super important. It helps doctors figure out why some people get this type of cancer and, more importantly, how to treat it. It's like knowing which wire to cut to stop a bomb—once we know about the ALK problem, we can target it specifically.

Remember, your body is amazing and complex. Sometimes things go a bit haywire, but the more we understand about these mix-ups, the better we can help. Science is cool like that!

Now let's talk about **ALK Lung Cancer!**

CHAPTER 2

WHO GETS ALK-POSITIVE LUNG CANCER

A Friendly discussion on to Numbers and Risk Factors

Q) ALK-Positive Lung Cancer: Who's at Risk?

Let's us now try to understand about who tends to get ALK-positive lung cancer. It's like we're putting together a puzzle, looking at the pieces of who, how many, and why. Ready? Let's dive in!

Q) How Common Is It?

Imagine a big stadium full of people with lung cancer. If we look closely:

- About **3 to 5 people** out of every 100 would have ALK-positive lung cancer.

- That's not a lot, right? It's pretty rare, which is why it's so important to know about it!

So, the takeaway message is **ALK-positive lung cancer constitutes only about 5% of all NSCLC** cases,

Q) Who's More Likely to Get It?

Here's where it gets interesting. ALK-positive lung cancer doesn't follow the usual rules:

1. **Age Matters:**

- It's like ALK-positive lung cancer prefers the **younger crowd.**

- Most folks with this type are **under 55**.

- Think of it as the hipster of lung cancers—showing up in younger people more often.

2. **Gender Mix:**

- It's pretty equal opportunity—men and women get it about the same amount.

- But some studies **hint that women might get it slightly more often.**

3. **Smoking Habits:**

- Here's a **plot twist**–most people with ALK-positive lung cancer have **never smoked!**

- If they do smoke, they're usually **light smokers.**

4. **Family Ties:**

- Sometimes, **it runs in families**. If your relatives have had it, you might want to watch. So look out for genetic history.

5. **Race and Ethnicity:**

- It seems to be a bit more common in the East Asia populations.

- But remember, it can happen to anyone, regardless of background.

Q) Risk Factors: What's the Deal?

Now, this is where ALK-positive lung cancer is a bit of a rebel:

- Smoking: Unlike many lung cancers, **smoking isn't a big risk factor** here.

- Age: **Being younger** is more of a risk, which is pretty unusual for cancer.

- Genetics: Your genes play a big role, but we're still learning exactly how.

Q) The Typical ALK-Positive Patient

If we had to paint a picture of the "typical" person with ALK-positive lung cancer, it might look like this:

- A **young adult** (maybe in their 40s)

- Probably **never smoked, or smoked very little**

- Could be **male or female**

- Might have **Asian ancestry**

- Possibly have a **family history** of this type of cancer

But remember, these are just patterns. **ALK-positive lung cancer doesn't discriminate**–it can **affect anyone, any age and any gender.** We have seen ALK positive lung cancer in **elderly patients as well.**

Q) Why This Matters?

Knowing who's more likely to get ALK-positive lung cancer helps Oncologist a lot:

- They can look for it in **younger patients** who might otherwise be overlooked for lung cancer screening.

- It helps in **choosing the right tests and treatments.**

- It reminds us that anyone with lungs can get lung cancer, even if they've never smoked.

While **ALK-positive lung cancer is rare,** it's super important to know about it. It likes to break the rules of what we usually think about lung cancer. So, if you're worried, don't hesitate to chat with your doctor. Knowledge is power, especially when it comes to your health!

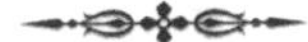

Chapter 3

ALK Gene Mutation and its Role in Prognosis and Treatment

Q) The ALK Gene Mutation: A Twist in the Cancer Story

Folks, hope you Remember how we talked about the **ALK gene getting mixed up** and causing trouble. Well, **let's dive deeper** into what this means for people with ALK-positive lung cancer. **It's like we're detectives**, and this gene mutation is our major clue!

Q) What's the Big Deal with This Mutation?

Imagine your body is a big city, and **genes are like traffic lights**. The ALK gene mutation is like a **traffic light stuck on green**. Cars (in this case, cells) keep going when they should stop. This **non-stop growth** is what we call cancer.

Q) How Does This Affect the Cancer's Behavior?

1. **Growth Speed:**

- ALK-positive cancer cells are like **kids hopped up on sugar**—they grow and divide super fast.

- This rapid growth can make the **cancer spread quickly if not caught early.**

2. **Spreading Habits:**

- These cancer cells love to travel. **They're like tourists** with **unlimited vacation days,** often spreading to the **brain and liver.**

Q) The Silver Lining: Treatment Options

Here's where things get exciting! Knowing about the ALK mutation is like **having the villain's playbook:**

1. Targeted Therapies:

- Scientists have created drugs that specifically **target the ALK mutation.**

- Think of these drugs as **special locks for that stuck green light**. They help slow down or stop the cancer growth.

2. Personalized Medicine:

- Doctors can now **tailor treatment** to your specific type of cancer.

- It's like having a **custom-made suit instead** of something off the rack—it fits better!

Q) What Does This Mean for Prognosis?

Prognosis is doctor-speak for "what to expect." **Here's the scoop:**

1. Generally Better Outlook:

- Thanks to **targeted therapies,** many people with ALK-positive lung cancer do **better than** those with other types of lung cancer.

- It's like having a GPS for your cancer journey–you know where you're going and have better tools to get there.

2. **Longer Survival Rates:**

- With the right treatment, many patients **live longer and better lives**.

- **We're talking years, not just months**, which is a big deal in the cancer world!

3. **Better Quality of Life:**

- Targeted therapies often **have fewer side effects** than traditional chemotherapy.

- It's like **taking a smooth road instead of a bumpy one**–the journey is easier.

Q) The Catch: Resistance Can Happen

Here's the tricky part–**cancer cells are sneaky:**

1. **Drug Resistance:**

- Sometimes, cancer cells **figure out how to bypass** the targeted therapy.

- It's like they've **found a secret passage** around our road-block.

2. **Ongoing Research:**

- Scientists are always **working on new drugs to overcome resistance.**

- Think of it as a **never-ending game of cat and mouse,** but we're getting better at being the cat!

Q) Why This Matters for You?

Knowing about the ALK mutation is super important:

1. **Early Testing:**

- Doctors can test for this mutation early on.

- It's like **checking the weather before a trip**–you know what to prepare for.

2. **Right Treatment, Right Time:**

- With this information, you get the most effective treatment from the start.

- No more one-size-fits-all approach–**it's all about what works best for you.**

3. **Hope and Progress:**

- The ALK mutation discovery has opened doors to **better treatments and outcomes.**

- It's a reminder that **science is always advancing**, giving us more reasons to be hopeful.

Remember, every cancer journey is unique. The ALK mutation might sound scary, but knowing about it actually **gives us more power to fight back**. It's turned a **tough battle into** a more **manageable one for many people. How cool is that?**

CHAPTER 4

SIGNS AND SYMPTOMS OF ALK POSITIVE LUNG CANCER

ALK-Positive Lung Cancer: The Sneaky Troublemaker's Calling Cards

Hey Folks! Let's talk about **how to spot ALK-positive lung cancer**. It's like we're learning to read the signs of a sneaky troublemaker in your body. Remember, your body is great at dropping hints when something's not right!

Q) What are the Usual Suspects: Common Symptoms

1. The Never-Ending Cough

Imagine a party guest who just **won't leave.** That's what this cough is like.

It sticks around for **weeks, maybe even months.**

Sometimes it brings an unwelcome friend: **blood**. If you see this, it's time to call the doctor, pronto!

2. **Breathing: From Marathon to Sprint:**

Your lungs usually work like a well-oiled machine. But now? It's like they're running a marathon they didn't train for.

You might find yourself **out of breath** just walking to the mailbox.

Stairs become your new Everest—challenging and leaving you gasping.

3. The **Incredible Shrinking Appetite:**

Food used to be your best friend, but now it's like an awkward acquaintance you avoid.

- Your favorite meals? They might as well be cardboard.

The scale starts showing lower numbers, but not in a good way.

4. The **energy vampire:**

- It's like something's secretly **unplugging your battery** every night.

- Getting out of bed feels like lifting a ton of bricks.

- Your get-up-and-go has got-up-and-went!

5. **Pain**: The Unwelcome Visitor:

- You might feel an ache in your **chest, back, or shoulders.**

- It's like someone's constantly poking you, and not in a playful way.

Q) The Plot Thickens: Less Common but Important Signs

1. **Voice Changes:**

- Suddenly, you sound like you've been to a rock concert every night.

- Your voice gets hoarse, like a frog has taken up residence in your throat.

2. **The Face and Arm Swelling Mystery:**

- It's like your body's playing a weird prank, making your face or arms puff up.

- This could be a sign the **troublemaker (cancer) is pressing** on some important blood vessels.

3. **The Eyelid Droop:**

- One of your eyelids decides to go on a permanent vacation, hanging lower than usual.

- It's like your eye is winking, but not in a fun way.

4. **Lumps**: The Bump in the Road:

- You might notice lumps popping up above your collarbone or in your neck.

- It's like unwanted speed bumps appearing on your skin highway.

Q The Plot Twist: Symptoms in Other Places

Remember, ALK-positive lung cancer **likes to travel**. So sometimes, the first signs show up in its **favorite vacation spots:**

1. **Brain Vacation:**

- **Headaches** become your new unwanted companion.

- You might feel **dizzy,** like you're on a perpetual merry-go-round.

- Your **coordination goes haywire**–suddenly, you're all thumbs!

2. **Liver Layover:**

- Your skin and eyes might take on a yellowish tint, like you're turning into a character from a cartoon.

- It's the cancer messing with your liver's normal operations.

Q) The Important Reminder

Here's the thing: these symptoms can be like **shape-shifters.** They **might pop up all at once, one at a time,** or some might not show up at all. And sometimes, they're caused by something totally different.

But here's the golden rule: If you notice any of these signs sticking around or ganging up on you, it's time to have a chat with your doctor. Think of it like calling a detective when you notice something fishy in your neighborhood. **Better safe than sorry, right?**

Remember, your body is pretty smart. It knows **how to wave red flags** when something's not right. All you need to do is pay attention and be ready to make that call. You've got this!

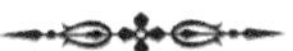

CHAPTER 5

DIAGNOSIS OF ALK POSITIVE LUNG CANCER

Imagine the Sherlock Holmes and the Case of ALK-Positive Lung Cancer

Hey there, **This is Oncologist, your health detective!** I am ready to solve the **mystery of ALK-positive** lung cancer. Let's put on our thinking caps and explore how doctors crack this case and save the day!

Who Should Be Tested for ALK-Positive?

The NCCN organization framed guidelines on who should be tested for an ALK mutation. The consensus was that all patients with advanced-stage adenocarcinoma should be tested for both ALK and other important lung mutations, irrespective of gender, smoking history, other risk factors, and race.

Patients diagnosed with lung cancer may have to be proactive in requesting molecular testing for lung cancer mutations. Some doctors are not familiar with the necessity of the tests. Again, your doctor may not understand the likelihood that you may have an oncogene-related (dna-mutation) cancer. Many, or perhaps most, insurance companies cover these tests. Your treatment plan and outcome depends on an accurate diagnosis, including genetic testing.

Part 1: The Investigation (Diagnosis)

Diagnosing ALK-positive lung cancer is like being a super-sleuth. Here's how doctors gather their clues:

1. The Interrogation (Medical History):

- Doctors play with multiple Questions about your health, habits, and family history.

- It's like creating your health autobiography!

2. The Stakeout (Physical Exam):

- Your doctor becomes Inspector Gadget, listening to your lungs and feeling for any suspicious lumps.

3. The Snapshot (Imaging Tests):

- **X-rays:** Like taking a black-and-white photo of your lungs.

- **CT scans:** Think of it as a 3D movie of your insides.

- **PET scans:** Imagine your body lit up like a Christmas tree, showing where the troublemakers are hiding. This determines **the exact stage** of the lung cancer.

4. The Smoking Gun (Biopsy):

- Doctors **snag a tiny piece** of the suspicious area.

- It's like collecting fingerprints from a crime scene.

5. The ALK Gene testing (ALK: The Villain)

- This is where **we find our culprit** - the ALK gene mutation.

- It's like **finding the villain's** secret identity!

Catching the ALK Villain: How Doctors Track It Down

Imagine '"**ALK**"' as a sneaky villain hiding in your cells, trying to cause chaos. To defeat this troublemaker, **doctors use some clever tools**—each with its own superpower to hunt down and expose the ALK villain. **Here's how the heroes do it:**

Part 2: Bringing Justice (Treatment)

1. **FISH (Fluorescence In Situ Hybridization)**: FISH is like a superhero. Think of this as a **magic flashlight** that shines on the cancer cells, helping doctors spot if the ALK gene has a special fusion. It's considered the **ultimate detective, the most trusted tool in the fight.**

2. **IHC (Immunohistochemistry)**: This hero throws a splash of bright paint on the cells, making the ALK villain light up so it can't hide. Itss a **handy sidekick to FISH** and gets the job done when needed.

3. **NGS (Next-Generation Sequencing)**: NGS is like

a **high-tech gadget** that scans every inch of the cancer's DNA, looking for the ALK villain and any of its sneaky allies (other mutations). **It digs deep and catches what others might miss.**

4. **PCR (Polymerase Chain Reaction)**: Think of PCR as a magnifying glass that zooms in on the tiniest bits of DNA to track the ALK villain's signature moves. Even the smallest clues can't escape its sharp eye!

Once we've cracked the case, **it's time to bring in the superheroes** to save the day. In the world of ALK-positive lung cancer, **our superheroes are called ALK inhibitors!**

The following are the superheroes in the form of ALK inhibitors:

- Crizotinib

- Ceritinib

- Alectinib

- Brigatinib

- Lorlatinib

Let us understand The League of Extraordinary ALK Inhibitors

1. Crizotinib (The Original Hero):

- The **first ALK inhibitor** on the scene

- Think of it as the **Superman of ALK inhibitors** - the one that started it all.

- It's like kryptonite for ALK-positive cancer cells.

2. Ceritinib (The Quick Learner):

- Came in when cancer cells started outsmarting Crizotinib.

- It's like the **Spider-Man of the group** - younger but with some fancy new tricks.

3. Alectinib (The Brain Protector):

- **This one's great at fighting cancer that's spread to the brain.**

- Think of it as **Professor X** - really good at tackling brain-related issues.

4. Brigatinib (The Flexible Fighter):

- May Work well even when other inhibitors have failed.

- It's like the **Shapeshifter** of the group - adaptable and resilient.

5. Lorlatinib (The Next-Gen Hero):

- The newest kid on the block, designed to **overcome resistance to other ALK inhibitors.**

- Think of it as **Iron Man** - constantly upgrading to tackle new challenges.

Q) How These Superheroes Work?

Imagine cancer cells are like **runaway cars with a stuck accelerator** (that's the ALK mutation). ALK inhibitors are like a super-mechanic that knows exactly how to unstick that accelerator. They zoom in and block the ALK protein, putting the brakes on cancer growth.

Q) How to design The Battle Plan?

1. First Line of Defense:

- Doctors usually start with **newer generation** ALK inhibitors, like **Alectinib.**

- It's like sending in your **strongest player first.**

2. Adapting to the Enemy:

- If one inhibitor stops working, they **switch to another.**

- It's like a **game of chess**, always thinking about two moves ahead.

3. Backup Troops:

- Sometimes, doctors mix in other treatments like:

- **Radiation:** Zapping cancer cells like a laser gun.

- **Immunotherapy:** Training your body's army (immune system) to fight cancer.

- **Chemotherapy:** The old reliable, like sending in a wrecking ball when needed.

4. The Victory Dance (Monitoring)

After treatment starts, doctors keep a close eye on things:

- **Regular scans**: Like satellite imagery tracking the villain's hideouts.

- **Blood tests**: Checking for clues in your bloodstream.

- **Symptom checks**: Making sure you're feeling like a super-hero should!

Q) The Ongoing Battle, How to Win?

Remember, fighting ALK-positive lung cancer is more like a **marathon than a sprint.** There might be **ups and downs**, but with these super treatments and your team of medical superheroes, you've got a fighting chance!

Always remember: **Every person's cancer journey is unique.** Your doctor will customize the **perfect superhero team** for your specific situation. And hey, **you're the real superhero in this story - stay strong, stay positive, and keep fighting the good fight!**

CHAPTER 6

SUPERHERO SHOWDOWN: COMPARING OUR ALK INHIBITOR CHAMPIONS

L et's have a **friendly competition** among our ALK inhibitor superheroes! We'll look at how they **stack up in three key areas**:

1. Progression-Free Survival (PFS): Think of this as how long our hero can keep the villain at bay.

2. Overall Response Rate (ORR): This is like the hero's success rate in defeating the bad guys.

3. Overall Survival: The big one - how long our heroes help people live!

Q) Lets analyze The Leaderboard Now

1. Alectinib (Our Brain Protector):

- **PFS:** Keeps cancer at bay for **about 3 years** on average. That's like **holding your breath for half an hour!** This makes Alectinib a **powerful and longer-lasting hero** compared to Crizotinib.

- **ORR:** Scores a whopping **83% success rate.** It's like getting **an A** on your cancer-fighting exam!

- **Brain Metastases: Reduces the risk by about 84%.** It's like having a force field around your brain!

2. Brigatinib (The Flexible Fighter or The multipurpose fighter)

- **PFS:** Holds the line for **about 24 months.** Not too shabby!

- **ORR:** Hits back with a **75% success rate.** Solid B+ performance!

- Especially good at tackling brain metastases that have outsmarted other treatments. Similar to Alectinib, It is strong and versatile, thereby defending both the body and brain from cancer spread.

3. Lorlatinib (The Next-Gen Hero And The Ultimate Brain Shield):

- **PFS:** As of the **CROWN study**, the **PFS benefit has not yet been** reached, **even at 5 years,** showing Lorlatinib's incredible long-term power in keeping cancer from progressing.

- **ORR: Around 70-80%, so it's highly effective** at shrinking tumors.

- **Brain Protection: Lorlatinib offers one of the best protections against brain metastases,** making it the **top choice** when cancer is in or likely to spread to the brain. Really good at shrinking brain tumors, with an **82% success rate** in the noggin.

4. Crizotinib (The Original Hero):

- **PFS:** Holds steady for about **10.9 months. Not bad for the old-timer!**

- **ORR:** Still packs a punch with a **74% success rate.**

- **While not as strong against brain metastases, it paved the way for our newer heroes.**

Q) What are The Resistance Movement: When Cancer Fights Back

Even superheroes face tough villains, and sometimes cancer cells learn to resist our ALK inhibitors. It's like the bad guys figuring out our heroes' weakness. Here's how it happens:

Q) Why Some ALK Villains Outsmart Treatment: Understanding Resistance?

When treating ALK-positive lung cancer, doctors sometimes face resistance—kind of like when a villain finds a way to escape from a trap.

Two types of resistance can make ALK inhibitors (the treatment) less effective:

1. **Intrinsic (or primary)**

2. **Acquired (or secondary)**

- **Intrinsic Resistance:** This is like the villain never being affected by the treatment in the first place—**it's rare,** but it happens. If the cancer continues to grow **within the first 3 months** of starting ALK therapy, doctors know the treatment isn't working. This happens in about **4%-10% of patients.**

- **Acquired Resistance:** This is more common and tricky. Imagine the ALK villain is caught at first, but over time, it learns how to escape the treatment and comes back stronger. This type of resistance **occurs after the treatment initially works well for a while. It's like the villains getting a new disguise that our heroes can't recognize.**

There are two ways the villain can escape:

1. ALK-dependent (On-Target) Resistance: The tumor still relies on ALK to grow, but it finds a way to dodge the treatment by changing its strategy.

2. ALK-independent (Off-Target) Resistance: This is when the tumor figures out an entirely new path to grow, using different "backup" routes that don't involve ALK at all. **Imagine the villains finding secret tunnels our heroes don't know about. It's like the bad guys installing super-powered fans to blow away our hero's attacks.**

The most common ALK resistance mutations are:

- **L1196M**: A common ALK resistance mutation

- **G1269A**: A common ALK resistance mutation that was resistant to crizotinib but disappeared after treatment with second-generation TKIs

- **G1202R**: A **common ALK resistance** mutation that is **frequently observed** after treatment with second-generation ALK-TKIs

Lorlatinib is a tyrosine kinase inhibitor (TKI) that is **effective against the G1202R** mutation in the ALK gene. It's also effective against other ALK mutations, including L1196M, F1174X, G1269A, and I1171X

Q) How to Outsmart the Resistance?

But don't worry! Our medical superheroes have tricks up their sleeves:

1. Switching Heroes:

- If one ALK inhibitor stops working, doctors can try another.

- It's like **tagging in a fresh superhero with new powers.**

2. Combo Attacks:

- Sometimes, combining ALK inhibitors with other treatments works best.

- Imagine our **ALK hero** teaming up with **Chemotherapy Man or Radiation Woman for a super-powered attack!**

3. Next-Gen Tech:

- Scientists are always working on new and improved ALK inhibitors.

- It's like our **heroes constantly upgrading their super-suits** to face new challenges.

4. Immunotherapy

5. ADC: Antibody-drug conjugates

Q) So, What is the Big Picture? It is the Overall Survival.

While our heroes are great at keeping cancer at bay, what everyone really wants to know is: **do they help people live longer?** The answer is a **resounding YES!**

- Patients on newer ALK inhibitors like **Alectinib and Lorlatinib are living longer** than ever before.

- Many are **surviving 5 years or more** after diagnosis, which is a big leap from just a few years ago.

- Our heroes aren't just winning battles, they're helping win the war!

Remember, every person's cancer journey is unique. These numbers are average, and your personal superhero story might be different. The most important thing is to work closely with your doctor-sidekick to find the best treatment plan for you.

Stay strong, keep fighting, and remember - you're the real superhero in this story!

Chapter 7

ALK Inhibitor Medications and Their Potential Challenges (Side Effects)

First Generation

1. Crizotinib (The Original Defender)

- **Vision challenges**: May cause blurry vision or double vision

- **Tummy troubles**: Might upset the stomach or change appetite

- **Energy depletion**: Can cause fatigue

- **Tingling discomfort**: Might cause strange sensations in hands and feet

Second Generation

1. Ceritinib (The Powerful Ally)

- **Digestive distress**: Can cause significant stomach upset (diarrhea, nausea)

- **Liver impact**: Might affect liver function

- **Heart rhythm changes**: Can alter heart rate

- **Blood sugar fluctuations**: Might increase blood sugar levels

- **Lung**: ILD/ pneumonitis

2. Alectinib (The Stealthy Helper)

- **Muscle discomfort**: Can cause muscle aches or weakness

- **Increased sun sensitivity**: Makes skin more reactive to sunlight

- **Weight changes**: Might lead to weight gain

- **Heart rate decrease**: Can slow down heart rate

- **Hepatotoxicity**: Liver damage

3. Brigatinib (The Lung Supporter)

- **Breathing difficulties**: Rarely can cause early onset breathing problems

- **Vision alterations**: Might affect eyesight

- **Muscle soreness**: Can cause muscle aches

- **Pancreas effects**: Occasionally impacts pancreas function

Third Generation

1. Lorlatinib (The Brain Barrier Crosser)

- **Cognitive fog**: Might cause confusion or memory issues

- **Emotional shifts**: Can affect mood

- **Hypercholesterolemia and HyperTriglyc-erdemia:** Might raise cholesterol and triglycerides levels

- **Speech difficulties**: Can make articulation challenging

Important Reminders:

1. **Only some people** experience all these side effects.

2. The intensity of **side effects can vary greatly** between individuals.

3. Always **report new or concerning symptoms** to your doctor promptly.

4. Your doctor **may adjust the dose or switch** medications if needed.

5. Some rare but serious side effects aren't listed here, so **stay vigilant and maintain** open communication with your healthcare team.

CHAPTER 8

ALK INHIBITOR INDICATIONS IN ALK-POSITIVE LUNG CANCER

1. The Early Skirmishes (Stage I-II)

- **Our regular body defenders (surgery and radiation) usually handle these small-scale threats.**

- **The ALK Inhibitor Superheroes are on standby, sometimes joining in special training missions (clinical trials) to prevent the villain from returning.**

- ALK inhibitors may be **considered in clinical trials** as adjuvant therapy after surgery in **high-risk patients.**

2. The Growing Threat (Stage III)

- The body requires strong defenders (chemotherapy, radiation, and surgery) to tackle this larger danger.

- If the villain leaves behind some henchmen or tries to return, the ALK Inhibitor Superheroes swoop in to clean up.

- ALK inhibitors **are not typically** the first-line treatment.

- **Standard care** often involves a combination of chemotherapy, radiation, and/or surgery.

3. The Big Battle (Stage IV)

- This is where our **ALK Inhibitor Superheroes truly shine**! They're **the first ones called to the** scene. ALK inhibitors are the **standard first-line treatment.**

- These superheroes **are more effective** and cause less collateral damage (side effects) than the old-school defenders (chemotherapy).

- As the villain evolves, we send in different ALK Inhibitor Superheroes with new powers to keep fighting.

4. The Villain's Return (Recurrent Disease)

- If the cancer villain reappears, showing the same weakness (ALK positivity), our **ALK Inhibitor Superheroes are quickly dispatched.**

- We choose which superhero to send based on past battles and the villain's new tricks.

The Mind Control Plot (Brain Metastases)

- Our newest ALK Inhibitor Superheroes (e.g., **Alectinib, Brigatinib, Lorlatinib**) have special powers to break through the villain's mind control barriers (blood-brain barrier).

- They're so good at this that they often handle the brain invasion on their own, without needing to call in the big guns (radiation).

Remember, every battle plan is customized. The superhero team (oncology team) works with each city (patient) to decide the best strategy, considering the body layout (patient's health) and the citizens' wishes (patient's preferences).

Q) Are there any Traditional therapies?

Traditional therapies such as **chemotherapy and radiation are less effective** than TKIs for ALK-positive lung cancer. Other new therapies, such as **immunotherapy, have not yet shown to work** better than TKIs in a first-line setting for ALK-positive non-small cell lung cancer.

Q) Do we have any Alternative and Adjunctive Treatments?

No alternative treatment has been tested and shown to be an effective treatment for ALK-positive cancer **by itself**. Please talk to your Medical Oncologist before adding any treatments other than ALK inhibitors.

CHAPTER 9

LIFE EXPECTANCY AND PROGNOSIS FOR ALK-POSITIVE LUNG CANCER PATIENTS

1. Outlook for ALK-positive patients has **significantly improved.**

2. Two decades ago, stage 4 NSCLC had **a 2% to 5% 5-year survival rate.**

3. ALK-positive lung cancer **responds well to TKI medications.**

4. Rapid **increases in patient life expectancy** have been observed.

5. A 2018 study found median survival for stage 4 ALK-positive lung cancer **was 6.8 years.**

6. Approximately **50% of patients lived longer than 6.8 years**.

7. Survival rates have increased since 2018 and continue to improve.

8. ALK Positive organization fundraises for research initiatives.

9. Significant funds are now raised for ALK-positive research

10. Ongoing research is expected to further improve survival rates.

CHAPTER 10

FINDING THE PERFECT ALK+ CARE TEAM

1. Finding your **perfect doctor** is like finding a **great teammate** - it's super important for your health journey!

2. Remember, even **ALK+ specialists** can have different skills and passions. It's okay to look for the best fit for you.

3. Reach out to the **ALK support group** - they're like a friendly neighborhood full of experienced folks ready to help.

4. Do some homework on your options, or ask a friend or family member to help if research isn't your thing.

5. Think of **hospital visits** like test-driving cars - try out 2-3 to see which feels right for you.

6. When you meet doctors, **it's okay to ask lots of questions.** They're there to help you feel comfortable and informed.

7. Don't feel stuck in your local hospital. If you're up for a bit of travel every few months, you might find a great match further away.

8. Ask about getting scans closer to home or travel help - there might be options to make things easier for you.

9. **Getting a second opinion** is always a good idea - it's like getting advice from two wise friends instead of just one.

10. Check out the **Second Opinion Program** - it's a great way to connect with top ALK doctors and feel confident about your care.

Remember, you're in charge of your health journey, and there are lots of people ready to support you along the way!

CHAPTER 11

COLLABORATING WITH YOUR HEALTHCARE TEAM

"Teaming Up for Your Health: Working with Your ALK+ Care Squad"

1. **Build a strong bond with your oncologist** - they're your cancer-fighting **partner!**

2. **Be open and honest** about how you're feeling and what you want from treatment.

3. **Don't be shy** - ask questions and speak up if something's not clear.

4. **Trust your doctor's expertise**, but remember your input is super valuable too.

5. **Share your emotions** - it's okay to feel worried or scared, and your team can help.

6. **Keep the conversation flowing** with all members of your healthcare team.

7. Stay curious about **new treatments and clinical trials** - your team can keep you in the loop.

8. **Be your own cheerleader** - advocate for the care you need and deserve.

9. **Learn about biomarker testing** and how it can personalize your treatment.

10. Remember, **you're the star player in your care team - your voice and choices matter!**

By working together with your healthcare team, you're creating a powerful alliance to tackle ALK+ lung cancer. You've got this, and your team has got you!

CHAPTER 12

RESOURCES FOR ALK-POSITIVE LUNG CANCER PATIENTS AND DOCTORS

Support Organizations for ALK-Positive Lung Cancer Patients

1. Support organizations are crucial for ALK-positive lung cancer patients.

2. These organizations provide resources, information, and emotional support.

3. ALK Positive organization offers educational materials, forums, and support groups.

4. Lung Cancer Alliance provides a helpline, events, and workshops.

5. Local support groups offer more intimate settings for connection.

6. Organizations advocate for increased awareness and research funding.

7. Resources include information on treatment options and clinical trials.

8. Financial assistance programs are available through some organizations.

9. Community events and fundraisers help raise awareness.

10. Support organizations help patients navigate their diagnosis and improve their quality of life.

CHAPTER 13

EDUCATIONAL MATERIALS FOR ALK-POSITIVE LUNG CANCER DOCTORS

1. Educational materials for doctors treating ALK-positive lung cancer:

- Overview of various treatment options

- Information on the latest clinical trials

- Knowledge of targeted therapies

- Understanding of prognosis and survival rates

- Importance of biomarker testing

2. Online communities for ALK-positive lung cancer patients and caregivers.

- Provide support and information sharing

- Allow discussion of treatment options and experiences

- Share information about clinical trials

- Focus on targeted therapies and genetic mutations

- Offer a platform for discussing prognosis and survival rates

3. Benefits of these resources:

- Keep doctors informed about the latest advancements

- Help develop personalized treatment plans

- Connect patients with similar experiences

- Facilitate information exchange between patients and doctors

- Improve patient advocacy and access to cutting-edge therapies

4. Importance of staying updated:

- Rapidly evolving field of oncology

- New treatment options constantly emerging

- Ongoing clinical trials advancing knowledge

5. Role of doctors:

- Provide expertise in online communities

- Guide patients through complex treatment decisions

- Stay informed to offer the best possible care

Conclusion

Summary of Key Points in the Comprehensive Guide for ALK-Positive Lung Cancer Patients and Doctors is as follows:

1. The guide emphasizes understanding ALK-positive lung cancer's unique characteristics.

2. Biomarker testing is crucial for identifying patients eligible for targeted therapies.

3. Early detection and personalized treatment can significantly improve outcomes.

4. The guide provides tips for patient self-advocacy and effective communication with healthcare providers.

5. Evidence-based recommendations are provided for doctors managing ALK-positive lung cancer.

6. Multidisciplinary care and collaboration among specialists is emphasized.

7. Ongoing research and clinical trials are advancing treatment options.

8. Targeted therapies, especially ALK inhibitors, play a significant role in treatment.

9. Personalized medicine through biomarker testing is a promising development.

10. Despite progress, continued research is needed to improve outcomes for ALK positive lung cancer patients.

REFERENCES

1. NCCN Guidelines

2. ESMO Guidelines

3. National Institute of Health

4. Devita, Textbook of Oncology

5. The International Association for the Study of Lung Cancer (IASLC)

6. National Cancer Institute

Websites:

https://www.jto.org/article/S1556-0864(15)32671-X/fullte
xt

https://www.survivornet.com/glossary/what-you-need-to-k
now-about-targeted-therapies

https://www.cancerresearchuk.org/about-cancer/causes-of
-cancer/inherited-cancer-genes-and-increased-cancer-risk/fa
mily-history-and-inherited-cancer-genes

https://newmobility.com/how-to-get-rid-of-epididymitis

https://www.alkpositive.org/what-is-alk

https://www.alkpositive.org/treatment-options

MAY I ASK YOU FOR A SMALL FAVOR?

I want to express my sincere gratitude for choosing to invest your time in reading this book. Your decision to explore this work among countless others means a lot to me.

I hope that within these pages, you've discovered actionable insights that can enhance your daily life. Your journey doesn't have to end here, though.

May I kindly request an additional 30 seconds of your valuable time?

Sharing your thoughts about the book through a review would be immensely appreciated. Your review serves as a beacon, guiding other readers to take a chance on my books. It's a small gesture that carries significant weight in the world of authors.

To submit your review effortlessly, please click on the link below. It will take you directly to the book's review page:

"Win The ALK-Positive Lung Cancer Fight"

Alternatively, you can also find the "**Reviews Section**" of this book's page on Amazon.

Your review will require just a minute of your time but will make a monumental difference in helping me connect with a broader audience and I eagerly look forward to reading your review.

Once again, thank you for your unwavering support of my work.

DISCLAIMER

This book is for educational purposes only. Readers acknowledge that the author does not render legal, financial, medical, or professional advice. The content within this book has been derived from various sources. Please consult a licensed professional before attempting any techniques outlined in this book.

By reading this document, the reader agrees that under no circumstances is the author responsible for any direct or indirect losses incurred as a result of the use of the information contained within this document, including but not limited to errors, omissions, or inaccuracies.

Adherence to all applicable laws and regulations, including international, federal, state, and local governing professional licensing, business practices, advertising, and all other jurisdictions, is the sole responsibility of the purchaser or reader.

Neither the author nor the publisher assumes any responsibility or liability whatsoever on behalf of the purchaser or reader of these materials. Any perceived slight of any individual or organization is purely unintentional.